The Break-Up

Your Lifeline Through the Absolute Dumpster Fire of Heartbreak

Kameron Matthews

Table of Contents

Thank you for reading "The Break Up - Your Lifeline Through the Absolute Dumpster Fire of Heartbreak!" If this book helps you navigate the tough waters of heartbreak, makes you laugh when you thought you couldn't, or simply reminds you that you're not alone, I'd be grateful if you'd share your experience with others. Your **Amazon review** could help someone else find the support they need during their own breakup journey. A few words about what resonated with you or how the book supported your healing would mean the world. Thank you for letting me be part of your story!

The Breakup Bible You Didn't Know You Needed

Welcome to a book designed to ease the emotional rollercoaster of a breakup. No matter what time it is or where life leads you, whether that be on the bathroom floor at 2 AM, stalking their social media profiles or simply feeling as though everything reminds you of them, this book can provide constant companionship in times of turmoil.

I understand what you're experiencing because I've been there myself. At 3 AM while sitting on my kitchen floor eating cereal out of its box and reflecting upon why someone could seem to change so quickly from saying forever one day and goodbye the next, my phone had died from all its social media updates; all my friends had gone to sleep; and all I wanted was someone to tell me I wasn't crazy for feeling as though my world had ended.

Once I realized this truth, I realized what every newly dumped person needs: an unwavering best friend who understands why you're searching "signs your ex misses you" at midnight; or why you keep their hoodie hidden away; someone who will know exactly what to say whether you feel strong or vulnerable.

This book can be your friend. It serves as an ever-present support system to turn to at any stage of a breakup, no matter where it may have begun. But be warned: breakups are messy affairs - emotions won't follow a straight path from sadness to healing; rather they'll shift back and forth rapidly as your mood fluctuates from sadness to healing - which is completely normal.

One day you might wake up believing you've accepted the breakup only to find yourself sobbing by lunchtime when hearing "your song." On another occasion, an ex could tag themselves in photos with someone new and cause further anger within you; just when you think things have calmed down further, bargaining with yourself promises of changing everything about yourself just so they return as your partner.

Emotional upheaval is an understandable part of grieving. In fact, it follows an established pattern known as the five stages of grief: denial, anger, bargaining depression and acceptance. Elisabeth Kubler-Ross first identified these stages in her groundbreaking book, "On Death and Dying", but have since been applied to all sorts of losses, such as breakups.

But here's the thing: grief's stages don't move in an orderly fashion; rather, they resemble an emotionally turbulent tangle with each emotion overlapping and interweaving with others. While you might pass through all five stages quickly or stay stuck at one for several weeks at a time - there is no set way or timeline for healing after grief has occurred.

That's where this book can help. Each chapter covers one of the five stages of grief with practical tips and plenty of validation to guide you through each stage. And unlike traditional self-help books which expect you to read from cover to cover in order to benefit, this one is designed so you can use it however best suits you!

Think of this book as your very own interactive guide to heartbreak: If you find yourself angry one morning, flip straight to the anger chapter for ways to channel that rage productively; if sobbing is part of your routine while grocery shopping due to seeing their favorite cereal, turn immediately to depression chapter; if things seem to have settled down since your breakup has taken hold of your life again and acceptance chapter offers support and advice about planning for the future - they all may offer useful tools!

But healing is an ongoing journey; just because you reach acceptance doesn't mean it won't arise again in some form or another. Grief is not linear and returning to earlier stages may occur as part of its journey.

That is why this book was designed to be used time and again when needed. Each chapter contains two parts, "THAT SUCKS" and "YOU GOT THIS," that are tailored specifically to help. The "THAT SUCKS" part aims at giving validation; we acknowledge just how painful a breakup can be and give you permission to feel everything you feel; whether that means sobbing into your ice cream cone or wondering whether you'll ever be able to listen to music without thinking of them again - these sections exist to say: "I understand, and it's okay."

But we don't want you to remain stuck in a state of misery forever. That is why the "YOU GOT THIS" section exists - as an opportunity to figure out what comes next and start moving in a positive direction even when things seem impossible. Here you'll find practical advice, pep talks and gentle nudges designed to get moving again when things seem impossible.

Unfollow your ex on social media so they're no longer constantly reminded of you; reach out for support when feeling alone; take a shower and put on clean sweatpants as small acts of self-care can sometimes make the biggest impact.

At its core, this book meets you where you are; it doesn't expect you to have all the answers or be able to "move on" from an ex overnight; healing can be a slow, frustrating journey that's best treated with kindness and understanding.

Use this book however it best fits into your needs - read it straight through from beginning to end, or pick and choose which chapter speaks to you right then and there, write in the margins, highlight parts that resonate and dog-ear pages you want to come back to later. Keep it by your bedside when 3 AM strikes or stash it in your bag so it's always within reach as a reminder that you aren't alone.

Keep this book in perspective: it is just a tool, not the cure-all you might expect it to be. Still, this book can provide validation, encouragement and practical advice to keep moving forward when things seem hopeless.

Because, let's face it, the world isn't coming to an end. I understand what you're feeling right now is intensely painful, and I won't minimize your experience of loss. Breakups are heartbreaking experiences; allow yourself to mourn what may have been and mourn for what could have been.

But I also know this: you are much stronger than you realize. Within you is the strength to not just survive this breakup but to thrive as well. Love again and build something even greater than what was before.

Your healing will not come quickly or easily; but with time, self-compassion, and the right tools (like this book!), you will make progress. One day you may realize the intensity of the pain has diminished; maybe you can look back without feeling like someone punched you in the gut? Plus you might rediscover parts of yourself that became lost during your relationship or create new dreams that are all your own!

I know this, because I've been there. My heart was broken into millions of pieces, and every inhale felt like an assault against my chest. Yet I also witnessed firsthand how even deepest wounds can heal with time and care.

As you embark on this healing journey, remember that you're not alone and accept that what you are feeling is valid; that it is okay not to feel okay sometimes; most importantly though, remember that you deserve love and happiness and that a breakup does not have to mean the end of your story.

This book is here to remind you of that fact every step of the way, serving as your three-am companion, pocket therapist and breakup survival guide. Use it however best suits you; each page turned will help bring you one step closer towards recovery from this painful period of your life.

Hearts have incredible resilience; no matter how broken they may seem. No matter how devastated or hopeless you may feel now, remember that no matter how broken you may feel right now you have incredible capacity for recovery, hope, and love again. Even when life seems hopeless at its worst - resilience, strength, and perseverance will enable you to build an even better life than before.

Your journey won't be straightforward or straightforward. Some days may feel like two steps forward and ten back; there will likely be moments when you question whether any progress has been made at all. Trust yourself and trust the process as each wave of emotion that passes over is creating strength and resilience within yourself.

One day, you'll look back and be astounded at how far you have come. Every moment of hardship was integral in shaping you into who you were always meant to become; therefore, this breakup wasn't the end but rather only just beginning of something great and beautiful in life!

Take a deep breath and let's begin our journey together. Whether you are deep in despair or just starting to see glimpses of hope - this book is here to guide, support, and remind you of your incredible strength.

Welcome to the start of an incredible journey! Now is the time for you to tell your own exciting tale.

Denial (Or, "This Isn't Happening Right?")

"We need to talk," came as an unexpected text message on a Tuesday or Wednesday - it all blends together after that three word statement appeared on my screen. I remember staring at my phone for several seconds while watching those typing bubbles appear and disappear, seemingly practicing how they'd break my heart apart.

Denial begins before someone even finishes leaving, when your mind starts making up possible outcomes while your world still disintegrates. Perhaps they want to discuss moving in together or planning an unexpected surprise; or it could simply be that what is happening is different than expected - your brain can be extraordinarily inventive when trying to protect itself from pain.

My mind spent an entire hour crafting intricate theories about what this conversation could possibly entail; each theory more hopeful than the last. By the time I sat across from them at our usual coffee shop, I'd convinced myself it wasn't a breakup; even our regular barista seemed concerned when their speech seemed foreign to my brain.

THAT SUCKS : During your first week apart from them, life takes place in a disorienting limbo: your mind works overtime to reject this new reality, and yet your brain carries on living normally despite itself. It's like watching a movie where both characters (you) are trying to change what will eventually unfold: when waking up you check your phone expecting there to be some sort of message saying they made an error in choosing you; before dressing for work with what to say when they call; finally going back over every conversation trying to identify hidden meanings or secret codes that might unlock an alternate ending.

Your mind does mental gymnastics as each word they say gets translated through your denial translator to sound like "see you later". "Space" becomes "temporary break." "Different directions" becomes "just confused". And anything "not working" becomes fixable by working harder - until eventually you begin speaking a whole new language that contains hidden messages of hope within every sentence spoken out loud.

Nights are tough; your mind often runs wild during those long, quiet hours between midnight and dawn, when every theory seems possible - be it testing love, dealing with personal issues, or just making up scenarios about why your partner might have left. Your own conspiracy theory workshop arises during those quiet hours where even outlandish explanations begin to seem reasonable.

As soon as your relationship starts to break down, things that would seem crazy a month ago become routine: driving past their apartment at midnight just to see if the lights are on; keeping their favorite snacks handy just in case they drop by; wearing perfume they once complimented in hopes that its scent might somehow reach across town; becoming adept at "accidental" run-ins that look suspiciously like military operations.

Social media becomes your own personal torture device. You become the full-time investigator of their digital life, examining every post as though writing a doctoral thesis on their emotional state. Every Instagram story becomes evidence. Every liked post becomes an indicator. Spotify playlists become secret coded messages for just you; can that sad song mean anything about us or was this workout playlist made specifically with us in mind?

Physical symptoms of denial are intense. Your body exists in an anxious state of anticipation: every door that opens could be them; every phone buzz could be their message; every turn could reveal their face. Your nervous system remains on high alert, waiting for that moment when alternate reality will become true: your hands tremble each time you check your phone; your heart races when you glimpse someone who looks similar from behind; your stomach sinks every time a text arrives from an unknown number.

Time slips away while we live in denial. Minutes can become hours while waiting for their response to casual texts you sent them; conversely, hours may quickly slip by while trying to remember hearing their voice again. Convincing yourself that time apart doesn't count is difficult when weeks can pass while remaining suspended in this belief - missing the reality that they have moved forward while you're stuck rewinding the story.

Denial sets in during bargaining, as negotiations for change become futile. Your brain begins devising elaborate IF/THEN scenarios in your head; convincing you that if only you could find the perfect combination of words and actions to bring order back into everything's sense.

Friends often try to offer support in different ways. Some enable your denial, letting you talk in circles about how this is all temporary or listen as you discuss theories like mercury being retrograde.

Others provide intervention-style tough love by showing dating app profiles or social media updates of those dating, yet neither approach proves effective; denial is emotional armor that protects us from facing harsh truths that our hearts cannot yet bear to face.

Your apartment becomes a museum of what-ifs: their toothbrush remains in its holder untouched; their coffee mug still sits where you keep it; their side of bed stays neat as though doing so might preserve a chance for their return; you cannot bring yourself to delete their shows from Netflix, nor remove their clothes from closet; each item becomes an emotional placeholder as you struggle against reality.

Dreams can be terrifyingly vivid. Every night, your subconscious creates scenarios in which everything works out for the best: reconciliation in coffee shops, airports and random street corners - they seem so real that waking up becomes heartbreaking - you take naps throughout the day, hoping to return to these alternate realities where they never left, while sometimes lying awake for hours trying to recreate these dreams or simply remain there where everything still feels possible.

Memory can be both comfort and torment. We replay every good moment, searching for proof that what happened wasn't real, while at the same time remembering things we ignored - such as how they pulled away when you needed them most, their plans never quite coming together, promises they made that always had conditions attached; yet our brain quickly dismisses these memories, determined to preserve a positive picture of your relationship.

Your job now becomes reading between the lines that don't even exist: their mom still watches your Instagram stories - an obvious sign she is on your side and pushing for reconciliation; their best friend views your LinkedIn update - perhaps they are checking up on them; while their cousin likes your tweet as evidence in your ongoing case for hope. Every digital interaction becomes evidence for you ongoing case.

As time passes, your world becomes divided into "safe" and "dangerous" zones: places you never went together; and coffee shops, restaurants and street corners that hold memories. You find yourself taking longer routes to work to avoid these landmines of memory; however, memories find you anyway: their song might play in a store aisle; their brand of cereal may sit on shelves; even strangers might wear perfume that reminds you of them - making the city a maze of triggers that require maneuvering carefully through.

Your phone becomes both lifeline and enemy as you devise intricate systems around texting them: wait three days; seem casual about texting back; draft and redraft messages until they come across as nonchalant as possible: "Hey, found your charger; thought you might need it" "Just saw that movie you mentioned; reminded me to check if we still have my copy of that book". Each text serves as an excuse to connect; each response (or lack thereof) scrutinized like it were code broken by the CIA.

Denial can be devastatingly real and powerfully dangerous. Your mind's way of creating an alternative reality that feels quite logical - such as "they'll come back once they realize what they've lost", "this will just pass" and that love like this doesn't just suddenly end - can all contribute to making denial so strong - yet dangerous.

YOU GOT THIS: Let's examine what's really going on inside of your brain right now. In response to overwhelming emotional pain, your mind creates alternative realities as a form of emotional morphine; dulling out sharp edges until you can bear them all on its own. No one here thinks you are insane; everyone makes mistakes. You are human!

First and foremost, creating enough distance from them is the first step to stabilizing your mind chemistry. Think of it like detox - although painful at times - necessary. Start with your phone - don't block them yet if that feels too painful, just mute their social media posts or chat history; archive chat history somewhere easily accessible but remove location sharing; archive photo files where accessing them requires extra effort; remove location sharing altogether from shared photos that might otherwise resurface easily.

Physical space is as essential as mental space. Even if you're not ready to give back their stuff or get back yours yet, we can create what I call a "Later Box." Put whatever hurts to look at in there such as their clothes or gifts from them as well as concert tickets you purchased for next month - not with the intent to dispose of them but simply out of daily sight line so as not to remind us too often of past hurts and disappointments. Your brain needs breaks from constant reminders.

Denial can be hard, yet its purpose can't be undermined; your mind's protection mechanism may just need time to work itself out. Just like entering a dark room requires time for your eyes and heart to adjust; acceptance shouldn't come rushing in; instead it must come gradually so as not to overwhelm or scare away its bearer.

Establish new pathways, both physically and figuratively. Try finding a different coffee shop, taking an alternative route to work or rearranging furniture - these small changes help your brain understand something is different from before. Don't focus on trying to erase memories - rather give yourself room to breathe without running into them constantly.

At 3 AM, the solution to your 3 AM problem lies within yourself. When lying awake and dreaming up elaborate reconciliation scenarios, something needs to break this cycle - not meditation apps or relaxing playlists; those can come later - right now you need distraction with purpose like cleaning out a drawer, writing down all thoughts that run through your mind, watching cooking shows or anything that occupy both mind and hands simultaneously.

No one warns us of denial's unpredictable nature: it comes in waves. At first you might experience moments of clarity where everything becomes evident before hours or days pass when all appears lost again. Don't see this as failure; think of it like learning to swim - sometimes you float, sometimes you sink; eventually though you figure out how to tread water successfully.

Your friends are concerned, yet don't understand why you can't simply accept reality. Show them this book, explain that denial isn't a choice at this time - it's part of how your psyche responds when threatened; ask them for support creating safe spaces where you don't have to pretend everything's fine; yet where they won't pressurize you into feeling better too soon.

Let's address the phone situation as it's likely the largest battlefield at present. Each notification makes your heart race, while every social media alert might seem related to this person. We must retrain your nervous system. In particular, change their text tone from something special like that which used to bring joy. Remove their contact photo - small changes which help your body understand that this person no longer forms part of daily life.

Establishing new rituals is crucial - not as an attempt to replace old ones, but in order to give your days structure that doesn't revolve around checking social media or driving by their apartment complex. Morning pages instead of morning texts. Evening walks instead of evening calls. Sunday self-care instead of brunches. You aren't trying to forget them - you are learning how to survive in an alien world.

Studies show the science behind what you're experiencing is real: romantic rejection activates similar brain regions as physical pain, making the pain all the more acute. Understanding this helps us be gentler with ourselves: just like someone with broken leg wouldn't expect themselves to run marathon, don't expect yourself to just "get over it".

Start paying attention to the small glimpses of reality that show themselves: whether it be going an hour without checking their social media, making plans without questioning whether they'll return, or simply deleting draft texts without sending. These moments don't represent failure but rather glimpses into your future self.

Let's establish a Reality Anchor System - not because you have accepted what happened completely, but to have something solid to cling onto when denial becomes too strong. Keep a list in your phone of facts - not emotions or hopes but hard facts like, "They chose to leave on [date]." Or they have stated they do not wish to try again." These simple statements will provide grounding when your imagination starts spinning elaborate reconciliation fantasies.

Writing can become your secret weapon in managing relationships. Beyond journaling, use writing as your secret weapon: write those texts you want to send but never will; discuss topics you wish you could have; write theories about why they left; get all those thoughts out of your head and onto paper where you can see them for what they are: your brain trying to make sense of chaos; writing helps move thoughts from emotional parts of the brain onto logical ones more quickly than speaking does.

Movement can be used as medicine. When denial strikes hard, getting your body moving - walking, jogging or dancing in your kitchen are great ways to remind yourself you're still here and still progressing forward even when life seems stuck - helps break free from mental loops of "what ifs." Physical motion breaks mental chains of "maybes" and "would-haves."

Denial's favorite lies: "They'll realize what they lost" and "This is only temporary". These thoughts aren't true - they are your brain's way of soothing itself - don't fight them; just label them for what they are and enjoy watching a movie without believing everything onscreen is reality.

As part of healing from denial, one of the hardest aspects is learning to live with uncertainty. Your brain craves concrete answers and wants a clear plan in place - this is why it creates elaborate scenarios to provide certainty where none exists. Learning to say, "I don't know why this happened" without quickly filling any blanks with theories is key for moving past denial and towards real healing.

Begin building what I call your "Self-Trust Fund." Every time you consciously choose yourself over denial, make a note. Every time you choose not to drive past their apartment or delete draft texts instead of sending them instead, acknowledge that decision as proof you're stronger than you think. These small moments add up and are proof you can stand strong against denial.

Reclaiming space takes time. Perhaps starting with sleeping on the middle of the bed instead of your usual side. Perhaps changing up your morning routine so you are no longer passing by the coffee shop where you used to meet. Perhaps creating new playlists without overanalyzing every song for hidden meaning is one step towards creating your new normal. Every small change adds up!

Your relationship with time needs to evolve. Right now, you are living in three time zones at once - the past where things were better, present where everything hurts, and future where you imagine them coming back. Practice living fully today rather than dwelling in maybes and what-ifs; living this way is exhausting!

Nobody seems to talk about it, but denial can be comforting in times of loss. That's why grieving can take time: slowly accepting they might never return while holding onto your belief they still love you can all help ease the transition between loss and acceptance. Each layer of denial serves its own purpose until we're strong enough to face reality head on.

Healing doesn't involve forcing yourself into acceptance; rather, it requires creating an environment in which both your pain and potential can coexist in harmony. Start small: Buy yourself flowers instead of waiting for someone else to send them; plan your month without leaving room for their return; choose something new to watch instead of binge watching "your" series; the more slowly but steadily you progress, the quicker you will recover.

Denial often takes form as a quiet transition, often sneaking up on us unexpectedly in quiet moments like making coffee one morning when you notice not checking your phone first thing, passing by their street without turning down it, hearing their song without feeling hopeful, etc. These signs that your brain is slowly accepting what your heart cannot yet comprehend aren't indicators that you have reached closure; they simply show how your brain has begun accepting what your heart refuses to hear yet.

One day, something shifts: whether it's seeing them with someone new, family unfollowing you on social media or finally reading their breakup text without the protection of denial, there comes an awakening and in its place is something new: anger.

Anger (Or, "I Hope You Step On a Lego")

THAT SUCKS: Your time in denial is up and it's finally time for anger - suddenly all love songs seem like nails on a chalkboard and every memory needs rewriting in ALL CAPS.

We've all been there - dreaming up petty revenge schemes, blaring Alanis Morissette to vent our emotions, and wondering whether or not now is an appropriate time to sign your ex up for cat facts texts. Anger after heartbreak can feel like taking an intense, slightly terrifying spin class taught by one of the Furies; leaving us questioning who we really are anymore.

Distress can quickly transform into self-improvement schemes when anger meets bargaining - often leading to early wakeups and juice cleanses - in hopes that once your perfect human specimen status has been reached your ex will realize they made a grave error in choosing you...right??

But here's the thing about anger - it can be sneaky. It often masquerades itself as justice or motivation and convinces us we are "telling it like it is" or not allowing them to get away with things; yet more often than not it just serves as an insulating blanket to prevent us from feeling what's underneath.

Consider this - when was the last time your rage spiral actually made you feel better in the long run? Sure, there may be temporary satisfaction in imagining your ex getting attacked by bees or falling down an open manhole; but these revenge fantasies only offer temporary highs; they don't nourish or support growth in any meaningful way.

And don't even get me started on social media stalking. We've all done it - obsessively refreshing our former partners' Instagram feeds in an attempt to decode every cryptic caption and "accidental" look-at-me-posts - but here's the thing: NO GOOD COMES FROM SOCIAL MEDIA STALKING; it's like playing emotional Russian Roulette: you may see something that makes you momentarily feel better or something that sends your blood pressure soaring; either way, it's a lose-lose situation either way - regardless of what happens.

But let's be real - sometimes anger feels good! There's a certain liberating force to channelling your inner Scorned person. Soon you find yourself striding down the street like in a music video, flipping off invisible haters and mouthing "I don't need you" out loud to nobody in particular. Perhaps this would make an excellent motivational speaker topic or self-help book entitled: "Thank U, Next: How I Turned My Breakup Into a Glow-Up."

Not to dampen your spirits; I understand anger can be an immensely motivating force - just look at every Hollywood post-breakup revenge body! However, eventually that anger is going to dissipate, leaving nothing but vague tweets and leather pants as reminders.

How can we manage our anger without spiralling completely out of control? How can we harness its flame without letting it consume our lives entirely? Buckle up - it's time for some honest discussion!

Anger after a breakup can be tricky to predict; it tends to come in waves that fluctuate with each passing moment, ranging from being completely fine and going about your day, to sobbing at a grocery store over seeing their cereal for sale. Just when you think you have it all under control, another trigger pops up out of nowhere and takes over your emotions once more.

As for triggers, post-breakup life can feel like one giant minefield of emotional tripwires - that restaurant where you had your first date? Trigger; that song that played when you kissed for the first time? Trigger. That cute inside joke that seemed cute at the time? Trigger!

Your brain seems to be constantly scanning your environment for anything that might remind you of an ex, and as soon as it does so, a surge of memories and emotions flood in, leaving you reeling with anger at every turn - often acting as the only buffer between complete disintegration and complete recovery.

But here's the thing - anger can be exhausting. Maintaining constant irritation takes an immense amount of energy. Carrying around an emotional backpack filled with rocks may feel great at first, but eventually your back and shoulders will feel the strain.

At this point, boundaries come in handy. They act like emotional scaffolding - helping you support the weight of anger without it collapsing in on you and provide a framework for dealing with feelings in an effective and sustainable manner.

What exactly does setting boundaries entail in practice? For starters, taking a temporary hiatus from social media might help set some clear boundaries. Although FOMO may be real, constantly checking an ex's Instagram story won't do anything positive for your mental health;

picking at it might feel satisfying in the moment but will likely leave an ugly scar behind in time.

Boundaries may involve creating some physical distance between you and your ex. This doesn't necessarily require moving to a different city or changing your phone number (though if that is what it takes, more power to you!), but simply being intentional about where and when you spend your time. Perhaps finding a different coffee shop to frequent or taking a different route to work would do.

Boundaries can also be emotional. This means making thoughtful choices regarding who and how much of your anger you share, as well as limiting its effect on conversations and interactions. Venting to friends or family is fine - indeed necessary! But there's a difference between processing feelings appropriately and constantly airing them out on those around you.

So how can you tell when venting has crossed over into toxic dumping? A helpful rule of thumb is the

"3-2-1" rule: for each angry, venting conversation you have, aim to have three positive, non-breakup related conversations; two self care activities and an act of generosity or kindness towards someone else.

The intention is that this exercise helps you maintain balance and perspective during a breakup. It serves as a reminder that even though this experience may be painful, there are other important things happening in your life and allows you to concentrate on those things which bring joy and fulfillment instead.

As for self-care - let's address it head on. In times of anger and heartbreak, it can be easy to neglect basic needs; before long you could be subsisting on a diet of anger-fuelled ice cream binges while staying up until 3am stalking your ex's Twitter feed and neglecting showering regularly.

Self-care should never be seen as optional; rather it should be treated like an essential necessity when going through something as difficult and distressful as a breakup.

So what exactly does self-care entail? At its core, self-care involves eating regularly and feeding your body nutritious foods that make you feel good; getting sufficient sleep - even if that means taking melatonin or listening to an inane podcast to shut out noise in your mind; moving in ways that feel joyful and energizing such as running, taking dance classes, or just stretching it out on your living room floor

Self-care involves surrounding yourself with people and activities that help you feel understood, supported, and secure. This could involve joining a support group, therapy sessions, or simply spending more time with those who uplift and make you laugh. Self-care means finding healthy outlets for any anger or pain such as journaling, artmaking or screaming into a pillow if needed.

Self-care means being kind to yourself. It means giving yourself permission to experience all your feelings without judgement or shame, while realizing that healing is not a linear journey with constant ups and downs or starting and stopping points along the way.

Reminding yourself over and over that you deserve love and happiness is the first step towards self-love and wellbeing, even if this relationship didn't pan out as expected. Looking at yourself in the mirror and saying out loud "I love you" even if it means breaking out in tears at first.

But here's the thing - anger isn't your enemy; it's an understandable and natural part of grieving that can help bring closure for what once meant so much to you.

The key is not allowing anger to consume you; the key is feeling and processing it before gradually letting it go over time, using it instead as fuel for personal growth and transformation rather than letting it consume you from within.

Yes, that may seem easier said than done; sometimes anger seems like the only thing holding you together - but trust me when I say there is life beyond this rage; love, laughter, joy and adventure await just around the corner!

Feel your emotions. Set boundaries. Take care of yourself. And most importantly, continue moving forward, day after day. Because not only are you surviving this breakup - but instead are thriving because of it, which is truly incredible.

YOU GOT THIS: Now that we've discussed the realities of anger management and healthy ways to channel it, let's move onto action steps to channel that anger into something positive and constructive. Here are a few ideas:

Writing an open and honest letter to your ex is an opportunity for self-exploration - this letter should never be sent, though! Use this space to get all your thoughts out on paper without feeling pressured into sharing them with anyone else. Be honest, raw and real as you express everything on paper before burning it or shredding into tiny pieces before disposing of it in some other manner - this exercise should only ever serve you, not them! This letter is for YOU - no one else!

Create a Breakup Playlist. Music can be an incredibly therapeutic tool, and nothing beats an angry breakup song to help you process emotions and take on life with renewed vigor. Gather together all the songs that make you feel powerful, rockstar, and ready to take on anything in life; blast that music at top volume while dancing around your living room like nobody is watching!

Engaging in physical contact sports such as boxing or kickboxing can be extremely cathartic - not only is it great exercise but you can meet like-minded individuals while venting your anger safely in an arena controlled by professionals. Plus it provides a fantastic workout and presents an opportunity to meet like-minded folks going through similar hardships!

Volunteer for a cause you care about. One way to channel anger and helplessness into something bigger than yourself is to find an issue or cause that resonates with you and dedicate some of your time and energy towards making a change - whether that means animal rights, environmental justice or social activism. By volunteering your time and energy towards making the world a better place while meeting like-minded individuals who can support and inspire you, volunteering will bring meaning into your life while providing an outlet.

Discover a new skill. If you've always dreamt of learning how to play guitar, learn French, or to make your own kombucha - now is the time! Plunging yourself into something new can help take your mind off your heartbreak while providing a sense of achievement and growth - plus it gives you an excuse to meet new people and expand your horizons!

Assemble all your courage for an exciting solo journey. A solo trip is the perfect opportunity to connect with yourself and gain some perspective in life, so book that flight ticket, pack your bags and embark on an adventure of your own making.

Whether it's a weekend escape to nearby city or month-long backpacking expedition across Europe; push yourself outside your comfort zone and discover just how strong, capable, and resilient you are.

Set up a gratitude practice. Yes, this may sound weird at first. But hear me out: when going through a breakup can make it easy to focus on all that's wrong in your life; by shifting focus onto things you are grateful for - no matter how small or insignificant they seem - your brain may learn to look for the good even during difficult moments. Start each day by writing down three things you are thankful for and watch how your perspective begins to shift gradually over time.

Remember, the purpose of therapy should not be to make things seem better when they're not, nor should you suppress anger or dull pain with drugs and substances; rather, it should provide healthy ways of channelling emotions while taking care of oneself at the same time.

At its core, this entire breakup process is about learning to love yourself despite what may feel like the world crumbling around you. It is about discovering your strength, resilience and inner rockstar; realizing you don't require anyone else's approval because you are whole, worthy and enough all on your own.

Continue to experience and process your feelings, setting boundaries and taking care of yourself while finding ways to channel anger into something beautiful and transformative.

Be mindful that this is only the start of something new - that each chapter you write on your own terms can lead to success and happiness.

Let's do this together, shall we? Together, you and I are going to get through this mess stronger, wiser, and more powerful than ever before. Let's do this thing together - together.

Bargaining (Or, "I'll Do Anything To Fix This")

Welcome to Bargaining Town, population you. Here, on the journey towards divorce or breakup, lies hope: you convince yourself that with just enough words, actions and grand gestures thrown at it from all directions you can undo everything that has transpired thus far and restore equilibrium to relationships as before.

Stay seated, this stage can be an incredible journey. Your mind seems to have turned into something between a used car salesman and hostage negotiator as you attempt to strike a deal with the universe to restore your old life.

THAT SUCKS: Let's start off by discussing the self-improvement bender. In this situation, one convinces themselves that by becoming their best version they will make their ex realize their mistake and run back into your arms. Before long they begin getting up early every morning to meditate and practice CrossFit; reading self-help books like they're the Holy Grail of relationship advice; all without success.

Make promises to yourself like "I'll be more patient", "I'll be less needy", or even just trying something new like hiking can make a big difference - maybe learning to love hiking will even bring back old flames! Once your flaws have been addressed, your former flame may see how much has changed and want you back.

Measuring your worth through how many self-help podcasts or gym visits is not really serving yourself; rather it may be done in response to some imagined version of your ex who may be watching and judging every move made towards self-betterment.

And don't forget about your apology tour: this is when you decide that just by saying sorry in an appropriate manner, your ex will forgive and things can return to normal. So you start crafting apology texts like they're Pulitzer-worthy speeches; practicing what to say when "accidentally" running into them at that coffee shop they love so much.

Apologies only work if there's something to apologize for; even then, they won't erase past transgressions; you can't apologize your way back into someone's life if they no longer wish for you there.

Assuming you haven't done so already, the grand gesture phase involves devising elaborate schemes to win back your ex, like some kind of romantic comedy protagonist. Perhaps showing up with a boombox full of all "your" songs at their workplace; booking a trip to Paris where you can meet at the Eiffel Tower; renting out billboards proclaiming your undying devotion are all possible scenarios that may help.

But here's the thing - grand gestures only work in movies; in real life they're more likely to get you arrested for stalking than bring back an ex. Even if they do work, do you really want someone who you had to convince to remain with you?

Bargaining is also the stage when you begin making deals with an external force. You might promise yourself to become a better person, volunteer more and never take love for granted again - or swear off dating altogether if the universe allows one more chance with them. When signs come your way such as songs on the radio featuring their name or billboards with their image and fortune cookies claiming "true love is waiting", convince yourself it all forms part of some grand design to bring you both back together again.

But unfortunately, the universe isn't like a vending machine where good deeds will magically result in relationships - even if that were possible, would you really want someone in your life simply because the universe ordained it so?

Bargaining can be tricky business. In reality, it's just another form of denial; you're still refusing to face reality while looking for loopholes and secret passageways that lead back to how things were before. Instead of moving forward with life as you know it, bargaining simply keeps us stuck and finding more creative ways of staying stuck.

As soon as you enter bargaining mode, the more likely it is that you will begin to disown yourself. Your focus may shift towards winning back your ex and away from yourself; your needs, desires, and dreams become secondary compared to theirs; rather than seeing yourself for who you truly are as an individual with inherent worth that should not need proving over time.

YOU GOT THIS: Relax. Although bargaining may feel like the only solution, I believe there's another route - one which leads to self-love, discovery and love without needing grand gestures or outside help to find success.

First and foremost, recognize bargaining as the coping mechanism it truly is - an attempt by your brain to regain control in situations that seem out of your hands and avoid feeling the pain of loss by convincing itself it can somehow undo itself.

But the reality is that you cannot control someone else's feelings or decisions; you cannot force someone to love you by becoming a better version of yourself, apologizing enough or making romantic gestures; even if it were possible, would it make you happy being with someone whom you had to force?

Instead of trying to control the situation, take control of your own narrative. Instead of viewing this breakup as evidence of failure or worthlessness, use it as an opportunity for growth and self-discovery.

Start by compiling a list of things you have always wanted to do but have put off due to your relationship. Perhaps travelling alone, taking dance classes, learning new languages or reconnecting with old friends are on this list - maybe volunteering for causes that matter to you or finally starting that side hustle you have been envisioning can also make an appearance on it!

Point being, find ways to bring joy and fulfillment into your life beyond simply looking to fill any void left by an ex-partner. Start seeing yourself as an entire being rather than half of an arrangement.

As bargaining thoughts arise, try reframing them. Instead of thinking "If I change these aspects about myself and then they'll accept me again", try thinking: "I deserve to be the best version of myself regardless of my relationship status."

Think differently: Instead of thinking, "If I apologize in the right way, they will forgive me and we'll get back together," focus on saying something like, "I'll apologize for my role in causing the relationship breakdown - not because I expect this action will change anything, but simply because I believe this action is the right thing to do.

And instead of thinking that "the universe will bring us back together if it's meant to be," try believing that you "trust in the power of life to bring me the love and happiness I deserve, whether with my ex or someone new."

As it's essential that we treat ourselves kindly during this process, it is also crucial that we are kind with ourselves during it. Bargaining can be exhausting emotionally and mentally. Allow yourself days where you simply wish to wallow in sadness or anger or frustration without exerting much energy - or moments where bargaining mode comes back into play even after having decided otherwise.

Recovering doesn't happen in a linear fashion - rather, it is more like dancing: taking steps forward and back, with lots of twists and dips along the way. What matters is keeping moving even if that means small steps every day.

Just keep this in mind - you are more than your relationship status! You are an incredible individual with many talents, passions and quirks of your own that offer much to the world as well as plenty of love to give and receive in return.

Don't allow this breakup to define you; don't allow it convince you that you aren't enough and must change who you are in order to find love again - you are enough just the way you are!

Please keep going, my friend. Every step counts and every moment counts towards finding ways to love yourself each day - even if that plan may differ from what you originally envisioned. Don't give up hope just yet - trust that life has something in store for you that you hadn't considered yet!

Believe in yourself and in your strength and resilience - because you really, truly do have this!

WAIT! THERE'S MORE: Yes, this may seem impossible at times - especially when your heart has been crushed underfoot - but hear me out - there are concrete things you can do to ease yourself through this bargaining stage with more dignity and less frowning.

First and foremost, let's address boundaries. While boundaries might not seem appealing in a post-breakup crisis, they're essential. Bargaining can quickly descend into begging; and beseeching can quickly evolve into "I have 27 voicemails from you and am considering a restraining order."

Setting yourself clear boundaries is of utmost importance when dealing with an ex. That might mean unfollowing them on social media (I know! it's terrible!) to avoid being bombarded by pictures of their new life without you; or setting limits for "accidentally" driving by their house each week; or setting yourself an acceptable cyberstalking time limit of midnight at most; 3 AM being too extreme).

As stated before, it's essential that you create some structure for yourself so that bargaining doesn't consume your life entirely - there's so much more you have to offer the world than being just another ex-partner or ex-spouse!

Another way of creating an effective solution is creating a "bargaining jar." Here, you can write down all the bargaining thoughts that pop into your head - you know, the ones starting "If only I had...," "Maybe if I just...", and "I swear I'll never..." Write them on pieces of paper folded up tightly before placing in the jar - once every week or when your jar becomes uncomfortably full take out each slip of paper from it and read it out loud to yourself -

Though it might sound counterproductive, actually visualizing your bargaining thoughts in physical form is powerfully transformative. It helps you recognize just how much of your mental energy you're expending trying to change or control past or future events and can reveal patterns in your thinking like whether you tend to blame yourself for relationship breakup or make grandiose promises to the universe in exchange for another chance at love.

At this stage, it's important not to judge yourself for these thoughts - they are an inevitable part of grief. Instead, the objective should be simply becoming aware of them so you can start gently redirecting your energy in more constructive directions.

Which brings me to my next point - finding healthy distractions. No, I don't mean drowning your sorrows with alcohol or rushing into relationships with strangers from Tinder (although no judgment if that's how it plays out - we have all been there). Instead, find activities that bring joy and fulfillment while reminding you who you are outside your relationship.

Don't be shy to lean on your support system during this difficult time. I know it can be tempting to isolate yourself when feeling heartbroken and ashamed (because bargaining may not be your crowning achievement), but your friends and family care about you, so they want to be there even if that means listening to you rehash an old story or watching you devour an entire pint of Ben & Jerry's in one sitting!

Reach out and communicate your needs; whether that's someone to cry with, help managing thoughts that arise during difficult moments, or remind you how awesome you are. If your support system is weak or nonexistent, consider consulting a therapist or joining an online support group designed for people going through breakups as sometimes admitting you need extra assistance can be courageous itself.

So there you have it, my friend: an overview of navigating the bargaining stage of a breakup. While it won't always be easy and there will certainly be times when you feel like giving up and asking your ex back in, trusting this journey and opening yourself up to love and joy lies ahead - only you must trust yourself enough to embark upon it!

Keep going forward; put one foot in front of the other; remind yourself of your worth and value even on days when it seems distant; hold onto hope - not necessarily hope of reconciliation with your ex, but hope of creating an amazing future that surpasses all of your original plans.

Because, you're amazing and someday someone is going to realize this and love and appreciate who exactly who you are - flaws, quirks and all! And when that day arrives, you will recognize all your struggle was worthwhile as it led you down a path toward love and happiness that was well worth the fight.

Keep going, warrior. I have your back every step of the way.

Depression (Or, "I'll Never Be Happy Again")

Welcome to Depression Town. When travelling through your breakup grief journey, depression will often feel like that stretch of barren desert where all booze has run out and all you can hear are your own thoughts playing over the intercom. Congratulations if you have arrived at the "sweatpants and ice cream" phase of healing; prepare yourself for an arduous journey ahead.

THAT SUCKS: Before we go any further, let us acknowledge the unpleasant reality that depression post-breakup can be. It goes beyond feeling down or watching The Notebook on repeat while crying into your ice cream (although no judgment if that's your process). Instead, it involves soul-crushing despair that can make getting out of bed feel like climbing Mount Everest with flip flops on.

Depression has a way of turning everything dull and grey. Everything that once brought you joy - hobbies, friendships and even bacon! - suddenly seems less appealing than before. Your motivation has taken leave of you; energy levels are subpar; self-esteem? Well...let's just say you don't stand a chance against superheros right now.

Sobbing. Your tears seem determined to turn you into an inconsolable human sprinkler system. Crying is everywhere: in the shower, car ride home from an argumentative meeting with your ex, grocery store when they see their favorite cereal; basically any flat surface becomes an excuse for you to sob your way out of a confrontational conversation with your ex partner...

Depression lies. Like that mean kid from high school who convinced you you would never amount to anything and would die alone with cats (not that this is necessarily bad!), depression tells you you will never be happy again and are unlovable, suggesting it might be best just giving up now and living a life of Netflix and microwave dinners alone. Depression has a way of rendering everything seemingly hopeless and hopelessly dismal, like you're stuck in an endless tunnel of despair without an escape route. Depression may prompt you to question every aspect of yourself - your worth, choices and very existence; making you question all aspects of your relationship and believe you could have done things differently; ultimately leading you down a path of self-loathing believing you are somehow fundamentally flawed and undeserving of love.

Let's also address the physical toll depression can take. Depression doesn't just involve emotional exhaustion - although that certainly is a part of it - but may also manifest physically in terms of headaches, stomachaches or an overall compromised immune system - it seems as though your body itself is rejecting any attempt at moving forward.

Your sleep might become irregular or nonexistent; your appetite might diminish or you could find yourself engaging in emotional eating binges; self-care may seem impossible: showering, brushing teeth and changing out of sweatpants worn for three consecutive days seem so ineffectual and pointless.

Depression makes you feel isolated even in a sea of people who love you; you might feel alone even when surrounded by loved ones who understand. Social situations that once brought pleasure may become burdensome or exhausting; leading you to decline invitations altogether and retreat into yourself even further.

As soon as you start isolating yourself from others, depression often follows suit and increases. Once in this dark place, there may appear no way out and escape is no longer an option.

Yes, everyone keeps telling you that time heals all wounds, this too shall pass, and that keeping active and remaining positive are keys to recovery from depression - but when you're struggling with the reality of depression it can feel like insult to injury; its timeline doesn't work like that of other illnesses or anything like that; you just can't snap your fingers and instantly feel better no matter how hard you might wish it were possible.

Finding the strength to continue can be an uphill battle; every fiber of your being tells you it's time to stop fighting, yet somehow the battle wages on. It can be exhausting and demoralizing - easy enough to believe this is now your normal!

But here is what I need you to hear, even if it means resisting it: this is not forever. Though the pain seems endless and insurmountable at this moment, there is light at the end of this tunnel; you will not feel this way for too much longer.

YOU GOT THIS: When it comes to post-breakup depression, remember this: you are definitely not alone. In fact, if there was a club for people experiencing these emotions and depression, lines would surely snake around the block (with dress up clothes optional but staining acceptable - including tears and ice cream stains!).

As it turns out, what you are experiencing now is both common and a necessary part of growing. From wisdom teeth removal to receiving your first parking ticket - painful experiences all share similar symptoms - people have been where you are right now: curled into their fetal positions questioning whether life will ever feel normal again.

They managed to come through it. And so will you! Although it may feel impossible now, when simply getting through each day is like wading through emotional quicksand, but rest assured, this is not the end of your story.

Your resilience, grit and sheer stubbornness are stronger than you realize. Consider all of the challenges you've overcome throughout your life - when it seemed as though there was no hope - yet somehow found a way. Breakups may seem unbearable but are far from insurmountable - with resilience, grit and sheer stubbornness you will come through this.

How can you begin climbing out of depression's pit? By taking it one day (or hour, or minute) at a time. Baby steps!

Be gentle with yourself first and foremost. Don't set unrealistic goals of productivity or positivity at this time; even if the biggest accomplishment today was taking a shower and zipping up pants is reason to celebrate; simply enjoy every small victory along the way.

Self-care is also important during this stage, and I don't just mean indulging wine and bubble baths (though those can certainly help). Instead, it includes more basic measures: eating regularly, staying hydrated, moving your body in whatever way feels good (even if that means just taking a stroll around the block), getting enough rest - you know all those essential tasks necessary for human functioning!

Reaching out for support can also be essential. Talking to others may feel daunting when suffering from depression, but isolating yourself only leads to further despair. Even sending an text message letting friends and family members know you're struggling can make an immense difference in how your situation unfolds.

If your usual support system is no longer providing enough comfort or you fear you might be heading down an increasingly serious path, seek professional assistance. Therapy can be invaluable when navigating the uncharted waters of heartbreak; admitting that extra help might be needed is one of the bravest actions possible.

Allowing yourself to express your emotions can also be of great assistance. I know, it may sound counterintuitive: why would anyone want to intensify the pain when everything hurts so much already? But trying to suppress or ignore emotions only gives them more power; trying to hold off feels is like trying to hold a beach ball underwater for too long: eventually it will burst through, likely hitting you right between the eyes in the process.

Allow yourself to cry. Scream into a pillow. Write angry letters that won't reach their intended recipients. Feel the sadness, anger, fear and loneliness...it all has its place here - not pleasant but essential for moving forward with life.

As you process your emotions, remember to show some self-compassion. Treat yourself like you would any close friend experiencing difficulty; remind yourself that you're doing the best you can, that struggles are natural, and that your pain deserves acknowledgement and care. Be kind and show kindness - especially on days you feel less like it deserves it.

Creative expression can also be therapeutic; whether that means journaling about emotions or creating art to represent how they're feeling or writing poetry that might make others cringe later (but remember: you always have the "delete" button available!), just find an outlet for all those big, overwhelming feelings you're harboring inside you.

Allow yourself a little fun, too. While the idea of having fun when feeling down may seem improbable, consider this: fun doesn't necessarily have to mean going out and partying all night or taking an extravagant vacation (though if that is what works for you). Sometimes all it takes to have some fun is watching an entertaining film that makes you laugh, taking a long bubble bath with a book you enjoy or baking cookies just because.

Finding small moments of happiness each day - even if it seems forced at first - is key for fighting depression, because depression doesn't just involve feeling sad all of the time; it also involves losing interest in what used to bring you pleasure. By deliberately seeking out experiences that make you feel good - even for just a brief period - you send a powerful signal to your brain that there is still joy out there in this world.

Keep hope alive even when it feels impossible. Remind yourself that this state is temporary, even though it might not feel that way right now. Grab onto those moments of light no matter how fleeting they may seem; they are proof that beauty and joy still exist even amid overwhelming pain - reminders that this dark chapter won't define your story forever.

And on days that seem hopeless and despair-inducing...that is when self-love becomes truly radical. Even when every fiber of your being urges you to give up...it is important that we choose ourselves over and over even though it seems difficult.

I know I keep repeating myself but healing is not a linear process. Some days may feel like progress has been made; on others it could feel like you're back at square one with despair overwhelming you again. That is perfectly normal and does not indicate failure - simply that it is human.

It's essential that we continue our journey even when it appears impossible, reaching out for assistance when needed, being kind to yourself during difficult days, finding ways to make life worthwhile again and most of all trusting that we will come through this.

Because here's the thing - you are so much more than your suffering, this one chapter of your story and this moment in time. There is love, light and strength within you even if it can't yet be seen by you.

Even in its devastating wake, this breakup doesn't define who you are; rather it serves as an important chapter of your journey - an experience which is painful, heart-wrenching and emotionally draining in its own way; but also one which has helped mold, teach and expand you in ways you never anticipated before.

One day - perhaps today or tomorrow, but in due time - you will look back on this time as it truly was: not an ending but the beginning of something exciting new in your life.

Right now it may be difficult to envision yourself as someone else; your mind might be telling you it's impossible, that this pain won't go away anytime soon, that this pain will stay put forever. I know this all can seem impossible.

But I am here to tell you, with absolute conviction, it won't. You will recover from this experience, find joy again, and love and be loved back in return.

As for me, in the meantime, I hope that you can find ways to be gentle with yourself: honor your pain while continuing onward, reach out for support when everything inside wants you to isolate, believe in your resilience even on days when it doesn't feel that way.

You've got this. Even when it feels as though everything has crumbled around you and life seems impossible... you have this. Take it one day at a time... just breathe through each hour until the day is done.

Keep going. Keep fighting. Take time out for yourself even on days that seem impossible. Choose yourself.

You are an incredible survivor and warrior; admire everything you've accomplished thus far in life, especially all your beautiful accomplishments after heartbreak. And I cannot wait for you to see all that lies ahead for you!

Acceptance (Or, "I'm Going To Be Ok")

Welcome to the final stage of breakup grief: acceptance. This moment marks when you finally begin to feel more like yourself again; your future no longer seems so dim, and you begin embracing the idea of moving forward with life. However, reaching acceptance won't come easily: it is often an arduous journey filled with surprises and roadblocks along the way.

THAT SUCKS: Acceptance does not mean forgetting or pretending the relationship never existed, nor does it equate with "getting over it," nor being without any sadness, anger, or hurt again. Instead, acceptance involves learning how to coexist with these feelings while giving space for them without letting them control your life - moving forward even though part of you might still look backward.

Moving on can be scary. Your ex has likely been an integral part of your life for an extended period, acting as both partner and best friend. Losing them feels like losing part of yourself; now it's up to you to figure out how to navigate life without them - while facing uncertainty regarding whether there will ever be anyone else around or if this time could be your last attempt at romance.

Fears associated with ending relationships are real but unwarranted; just because one relationship ended doesn't mean you must settle into an isolated life of solitude. There are billions of people out there to meet, increasing your odds of finding another person to share your life with. Yet before diving headfirst into another one, important work needs to be completed on yourself first - something new a relationship shouldn't replace.

Journeying towards acceptance often means confronting "firsts," like your first birthday without them or holiday without them or anniversary of your split up. These milestones may feel like emotional landmines that threaten to undo all your hard work toward accepting this loss and may feel as though the universe is testing you to see if you truly accept what has occurred.

Acceptance can be uncomfortable at first, but every small victory made is progress towards acceptance. Every time you allow yourself to feel your emotions without judgment, choose self-care over destruction, and persevere despite pain, you are winning small battles toward lasting acceptance that gradually become part of everyday life.

Returning to dating can be an exhilarating journey, full of hope and anticipation only to encounter harsh realities like ghosting, breadcrumbing and situationships. Even when you do meet someone special again, it can be hard not to compare them against their past partners; constantly measuring potential new love interests against your old.

Comparison is detrimental. Every person and relationship is unique, so trying to recreate past experiences will only end in disappointment and frustration. Acceptance means learning to appreciate people for who they are now instead of who you wish they could become in the future.

At its core, acceptance means showing appreciation for what your past relationship taught you - no matter how painfully. It means acknowledging your strength and resilience through each stage of grief recovery; accepting changes as they come and opening your heart up to new experiences, adventures, or love even if it looks different than before.

YOU GOT THIS: So how can you reach acceptance, transition from simply surviving to thriving and transform your life for the better? It all starts with self-love.

Self-love is often disregarded as an irrelevant or hippie-dippy concept. Yet self-love should be the cornerstone of acceptance - and the basis for building an authentic, fulfilling, and joyful life without needing someone else as your partner.

Self-love means showing yourself kindness, compassion, and respect as you would do for a dear friend. It includes setting healthy boundaries, learning to say no when something doesn't serve your goals, prioritizing your needs over those of others, even when this means disappointing someone else from time to time.

Self-love involves forgiving oneself for any perceived shortcomings or mistakes. While it is easy to blame yourself for an unpleasant breakup or punish yourself for taking too long to "get over it", forgiveness is key component of acceptance; extend yourself the same grace and compassion that you would offer anyone else going through a challenging period.

Another integral aspect of self-love is learning to trust yourself again after experiencing heartache in relationships. After such experiences, it can be tempting to question every decision and wonder whether something's broken inside yourself that no one else sees or loves. But true acceptance means having faith in your intuition, resilience and the capacity for creating a beautiful life on your terms.

Start small. Make decisions that feel good to you, even if they may not make sense to anyone else. Surround yourself with people and activities that give your soul meaning; cultivate curiosity and adventure while remaining open to new experiences as they arise; be open-minded towards new possibilities!

Above all else, cultivate gratitude - not only for big gifts that bring us happiness; also be thankful for small, everyday blessings that add meaning and make life worthwhile. These moments remind us of life's beauty even in times of hardship or uncertainty.

Like the rest of this process, acceptance isn't always linear. There may be times when it feels like you're back at square one and your grief feels fresh and raw again; moments where everything seems off and questions if you will truly find happiness again arise; yet these aren't signs of failure but progress;

these moments remind us healing is not a destination but an ongoing journey that requires patience, self-compassion, and showing up even when difficult.

As you practice acceptance - choosing self-love over self-hatred, trusting yourself to make decisions that align with your values and desires, opening yourself up to new possibilities and adventures - it becomes easier and feels like home more quickly.

Acceptance is about reconnecting with yourself, the person who was meant to be before heartache, grief and pain forced you into hiding. It means coming home to an authentic, fulfilling and joyful life not because someone else is there but because you have yourself as your muse.

Do not hesitate to take steps forward even when the way ahead seems uncertain or when choosing yourself may feel selfish or frightening. Keep opening yourself up to all of life's beauty, even when the temptation may arise to close off and retreat into yourself.

You are worthy of love, happiness, and joy. You possess the tools necessary to build a life that makes your soul come alive and are prepared to embark upon the next chapter in your story - one which you have written yourself while remaining guided by heart and head.

I hope when you look back on this time in your life - the agony, heartache, and despair which once gripped you - you will recognize it not as a defeat but as an opportunity for transformation: as an opportunity to love yourself more deeply than ever before while trusting in your strength, resilience, and worth.

At its heart, acceptance is a transformative act that brings beauty, power, and hope into our lives.

Navigating the road to acceptance can be challenging, particularly if your heart feels as if it has been ground into dust. But there are steps you can take to help navigate through this stage more gracefully and less facepalm-inducingly.

Let's first discuss boundaries. Boundaries might not be your favorite topic when dealing with post-breakup angst, but they're essential. Acceptance quickly turns to begging; then comes "I have 27 voicemails from you and am considering filing a restraining order."

Establish clear boundaries for yourself. This could involve unfollowing your ex on social media so they're no longer bombarding you with photos from their new life without you; setting limits on how often you "accidentally" drive by their house each week; setting a curfew for late-night cyberstalking sessions - or anything else to establish structure so acceptance doesn't consume your entire life! Remember, you have so much more to give the world than being an ex-partner!

Another effective tool is an acceptance jar. Every time your thoughts include phrases like, "If only I had...", "Maybe if I just...", or "I swear I'll never..." write them out on paper slips and drop them in your jar. Every week (or whenever your jar becomes overflowing), take out all the slips of paper and read them aloud to yourself as an activity to unburden yourself of any unnecessary burdens.

Visualizing your acceptance-related thoughts in physical form can be powerful. It helps you realize how much energy is spent trying to alter past events or control future ones, as well as any patterns in your thinking - such as attributing blame for relationship breakdown to yourself or making grandiose promises in exchange for another chance at life.

At this stage, it is not necessary to judge yourself for these thoughts - they are an unavoidable part of grief. Instead, awareness should increase so you can gently redirect energy towards something more productive.

Finding healthy distractions is crucial. This doesn't mean numbing out with alcohol or engaging in risky behavior - instead focus on activities that bring you joy and fulfillment and can help rediscover who you are outside your relationship.

Start taking classes you've always wanted to, joining a sports league, volunteering at animal shelters or starting new hobbies that remind you of who you are - something that reminds you of your strength, creativity and resilience.

Don't be afraid to reach out for support during this difficult time as well. Support is valuable no matter stage you are in. Acceptance can be isolating, so it may be tempting to withdraw into yourself in times of heartache and shame - but your friends and family love you and want to be there for you no matter if that means listening as you recount the same story over and over or witnessing you devour a whole cake in one sitting!

Reach out to your loved ones and express what is going on for you, whether that means someone to listen, a distraction from thoughts, or someone who reminds you how awesome you are. If your support system is lacking, consider joining a support group or seeking therapy - sometimes being honest is the bravest move of all!

Acceptance doesn't mean forgetting your ex or the relationship; rather, it means learning how to coexist with memories and emotions while creating space for new experiences and love. Acceptance involves acknowledging past hurts while welcoming the present with eager anticipation for what lies ahead in the future.

Your strength, courage and resilience will see you through this challenging period. Keep taking steps forward, choosing yourself and believing in your worth; acceptance may be challenging but can lead to a life of love, joy and endless possibilities.

Modern Dating in a Digital World: New Rules for New Fools in Love

Modern romance is an intriguing mix of Jane Austen meets Black Mirror; an intricate blend of old-fashioned courtship rituals and futuristic technology which would even leave George Orwell bewildered.

Welcome to the modern world, where ghosting, zombieing and breadcrumbing reign supreme - where your biggest threat to love may not be an ex or mother-in-law who wants their way but rather your social media addiction and pocket supercomputer you carry around every day.

Well, I get it; after experiencing the emotional equivalent of nuclear war, the last thing on your mind may be getting back into dating again. And who could blame you? After having had your heart torn out by someone new, the prospect of dating again seems as appealing as getting a root canal treatment by an intoxicated dentist. But take heart: there's still hope out there; just putting yourself out there won't kill anyone!

But here's the thing: whether or not it's easy, sooner or later you will want to test out modern love again - and when that time comes, be ready for all of its unique challenges (and opportunities). Dating online requires preparation.

First things first: Let's discuss ghosting. For those unfamiliar, ghosting occurs when a relationship suddenly dissipates without warning; no phone call, text message, smoke signal, or carrier pigeon communication from either party; just silence. And this leaves one with an unsettling sense that they were wrong about them being as awesome.

Ghosting is the dating equivalent of leaving an event without saying goodbye, and has become so common that there are even subcategories dedicated to it, such as "soft ghosting" (when someone slowly fades away) and "Caspering" (where someone ghosts you in an amicable fashion; apparently this has become an accepted practice).

If you've been ghosted, first of all I sincerely apologize - it hurts and it isn't your fault. Although it can be tempting to internalize this rejection and begin questioning yourself and self-worth, remember that ghosting says more about them than you. Anyone who would prefer not engaging in mature discussions about their emotions face-to-face is probably not someone worth spending time with in any case.

So how should you handle it? My best advice would be to resist the urge to reach out. While it can be tempting to send that "hey stranger" text or like their recent Instagram post just so they know you exist, donning this guise will only make matters worse over time - engaging with your ghost will only grant them more control over you emotionally.

Instead, surround yourself with people who make you feel good, engage in activities that bring joy and fulfillment, and remember that your worth does not depend on whether some emotionally stunted individual decides to send back texts back.

Consider ghosting as an opportunity when the time is right (but only then!). Think of ghosting as taking out your trash quickly and painlessly - an easy and quick way to rid your dating pool of those who are emotionally unavailable, commitment-phobic or simply rude.

Let's discuss digital-clean up. After a breakup, your online presence can become a source of painful reminders and potential awkwardness. There's the question of what to do with all those couple photos cluttering up Instagram feeds or shared Netflix accounts with all your ex's odd documentary preferences still visible on them, not to mention any trace left by Facebook of your relationship status change.

At the core, there's no single "right" way to handle your digital footprint post-breakup. Some may opt for the intensely purge every sign of their ex from their online life like performing an exorcism on an iPhone; others take a more measured and refined approach while untangling digital lives while still trying to maintain some sense of civility and maturity in their online interactions.

At the end of the day, it's up to you to decide what feels right for you; here are a few general guidelines:

Take your time. There's no rush to making decisions that could potentially have lasting repercussions, like deleting photos or unfriending mutual acquaintances. Give yourself time to process how you're feeling before rushing in with that "block" button as a weapon.

Communication with your ex may seem awkward now, but having a conversation with the person who just broke your heart may be essential if there are digital assets involved, such as sharing Netflix accounts or joint email accounts between yourselves. Establishing some ground rules early could save much discomfort later.

Be mindful of mutual friends. In today's age of social media, breakups can quickly turn volatile when both partners share connections. Before unfriending your former flame's second cousin twice-removed out of spite or to make your point clearer, take a step back to consider all potential fallout and consider whether creating drama or hurt feelings for no good purpose would really be worth the risk - sometimes taking the high road is best.

Once the dust has settled, take time to reclaim your digital identity as your own. Update your profile pictures, curate your feeds to reflect your new single status, and begin posting content that makes you feel good. Your digital life is an extension of real life; only you can decide how it shows up both places.

Let's turn our focus to what you have been waiting for: getting back out there. After experiencing heartbreak, the idea of opening yourself up to love may feel as unattractive as having your colonoscopy done again voluntarily. But the truth is: just because your last relationship ended in heartache doesn't mean your future holds nothing but Netflix binges and microwave meals for one.

Post-breakup periods can be invaluable moments of self-discovery and development - not to mention pure fun! But if you decide to re-enter dating waters after having experienced heartbreak or divorce, be wary and set your nonsense detector high.

First and foremost: take time for yourself. This involves processing your emotions, taking an honest inventory of yourself as a partner in this breakup, and getting clear on what kind of relationships best suit your individual needs and requirements. It may mean taking an extended hiatus from dating altogether in order to focus on personal growth and healing.

When it's time to begin swiping again, be deliberate about your approach. Don't just download Tinder because you're bored on a

Saturday night while all of your couple friends are busy doing couple stuff - really consider what type of experience you want; be that casual hookups, serious relationships or something in between; then select appropriate platforms and approaches accordingly.

Digital boundaries come in handy here. In a world where potential matches are just a swipe away, it can be tempting to jump headfirst into new relationships before being fully prepared - but just because someone appears attractive online doesn't mean they are suitable for you or can fulfill the relationship you envision for yourself.

Begin slowly. Don't feel pressured to move too quickly, and don't be afraid to set boundaries around communication, availability, and intimacy - after all, your love life belongs solely to you and what works for you is ultimately determined by what feels good to you.

And if you find yourself falling for someone new? Allow yourself to feel all of the emotions - but do so with an open mind. In today's digitized world, it can be easy to become consumed with fantasy relationships before meeting face to face; just because someone can send an engaging text or charm you on Instagram doesn't mean they will be an ideal partner in real life.

So take your time, trust your instincts, and don't be shy about asking for what you need. If someone refuses to meet halfway or respect your boundaries, that should serve as a red flag - no matter how many "heart eye emojis" they send your way.

Be reminded: dating should be enjoyable! While dating can be scary and vulnerable at times - and even frustrating - it should also be exhilarating and unexpected, full of possibilities and joy. Don't take dating too seriously: approach it with an open heart and sense of humor while trusting that the right person will come along when the time is right.

Focus your energy on falling in love with yourself first - date yourself. Take yourself out for fancy dinners and long beach walks; buy flowers and write love notes - treat yourself as you would treat a partner because, at the end of the day, the most significant relationship in your life is the one with yourself!

Who knows? Perhaps your next great romance will begin with a swipe right - or it could begin through serendipity from well-meaning friends, or through serendipity that seems too good to be true!

No matter where the story begins, remember this: no matter who or what starts it all off, remember this: you deserve love exactly as you are and are enough as an individual - no ghosting, breadcrumbing, or digital drama needed to tell it!

So venture forth into dating, you glorious digital-age dating warrior! May your swipes prove fruitful and your boundaries strong while remaining open to all possibilities that lay before you - and may you always, always swipe right on yourself first.

So venture forth into dating, you glorious digital-age dating warrior! May your swipes prove fruitful and your boundaries strong while remaining open to all possibilities that lay before you - and may you always, always swipe right on yourself first.

But before you dive headfirst into the dating pool, there's one more thing we need to address - that person from your past who might still be swimming in the same waters. You know who I'm talking about. Your ex. Because in our hyper-connected world, moving forward often means learning to navigate the space where your past and present collide.

The Ex Factor: Transforming Your Relationship with Your Ex

Let's address the elephant in the room: your former flame. Not their memory or Instagram pictures you still haven't deleted - rather, them as an actual living, breathing person who still exists somewhere out there and may show up in your life unexpectedly, such as an ads notification.

Moving on can be hard - sometimes not just physically but psychologically too. Associating with former partners can feel like trying to defuse an explosive device with one wrong move: all hell could break loose!

As you co-parent with them, there's the uncomfortable dance of small talk when running into each other at mutual friends' events, the internal debate of whether to wish them a happy birthday and complex calculations about whether you can attend concert, wedding or party if they might attend; then adding co-parenting complexities add an entirely different dynamic! When trying to coordinate schedules and make joint decisions with someone who used to be your partner - but now acts more as an associate laden with more emotional baggage than before!

Finding a balance can be a struggle, and finding it can often seem impossible. Too much friendliness could lead to familiar patterns being repeated or false hopes being offered up; too little warmth might come across as bitter or unprofessional - not to mention having to manage your emotions while maintaining appropriate boundaries.

Sometimes it seems as though your ex has developed an uncanny knack of knowing exactly when you need support, from showing up when you're having a good day to popping up just after therapy or sending "hope you're doing well" texts at just the moment when your guard has finally been let down.

There's also the matter of mutual friends - those unfortunate souls caught between your emotional combat royale. While doing their best to maintain relationships between both of you while preventing diplomatic incidents, mutual friends find themselves carefully crafting responses like "Oh, that's nice" when accidentally mentioning your ex's new job, house, or relationship - while internally screaming into nothingness.

Social media makes everything exponentially more complex. Making decisions such as blocking, unfollowing or muzzling their posts feels loaded with meaning; mutual friends will undoubtedly scrutinize whatever decision you make as though writing an academic thesis on post-breakup etiquette.

Never-ever expect the uncomfortable situation of "running into them with someone new" scenario to go smoothly; nothing quite prepares you for that awkward moment when your former flame appears with their new partner while shopping for toilet paper at Target in your old gym attire and you're expected to make polite conversation while your brain disassembles and the fight-or-flight response kicks in full gear.

At its core, having a relationship with an ex doesn't involve either being friends or enemies; it means being at peace with their existence in your world, even if that means sometimes crossing paths again. Focusing on creating healthy boundaries that work best for your unique situation.

When engaging with social circles that involve ex-encounters, creating what I call a "professional persona" for these interactions can be invaluable. Think of it as creating an alternate version of yourself who can navigate situations gracefully without engaging emotionally - this way pleasantries and necessary social interactions can take place without getting drawn into emotional turmoil that often ensues during such encounters.

Co-parenting can be challenging, so approaching interactions like business meetings can help maintain necessary distance and ensure effective communication about your children's needs. Utilizing co-parenting apps, documenting important conversations and setting clear boundaries around personal lives are all ways that co-parents can create an enduring dynamic that prioritizes children's well-being while not undermining emotional health.

Working in the same professional field with your ex requires careful manoeuvring. Focusing conversations only on work-related matters and creating a support network outside your shared workplace are all ways of keeping yourself safe if things become untenable - perhaps even considering career moves should things turn unpleasant.

The key to managing all these scenarios lies in shifting your perspective from emotional to strategic. Instead of seeing interactions with your ex as opportunities to create closure or reconnect, consider them neutral exchanges that require neither emotional investment or energy depletion - similar to dealing with an awkward neighbor, you politely interact but don't need to know too much about each other's lives or divulge too many personal details about yours.

Some general principles can help guide any interaction with an ex. To begin with, keep any greeting or interaction brief - three seconds or less should suffice - greeting them quickly with a neutral comment before moving on with your day. Only provide selective sharing of information; your former flame does not need to know all about your dating life, career moves or personal growth journey. Finally, create specific times and places to process feelings related to them such as therapy sessions, journal writing or talks with friends so that any potential conflict does not escalate during interactions themselves.

Establishing clear guidelines for yourself regarding what forms of interaction are and aren't acceptable can help maintain consistent boundaries. Enlisting help from specific friends during post-ex encounter debriefing sessions and emotional support may make these situations feel more manageable.

Never forget, it is perfectly normal to feel uncomfortable around an old flame; some days seeing your ex can feel like an emotional gut punch. The goal shouldn't be making best friends out of them but rather creating a sustainable dynamic which protects your peace.

To effectively change your relationship with an ex, consider altering how you perceive them. Instead of viewing them only as someone who caused hurtful experiences, consider looking at this relationship as a valuable teacher - what lessons did this relationship teach you about yourself, your boundaries, needs, and values? For every negative thought about an ex that arises, challenge yourself to find something positive from this encounter - this doesn't mean dismissing hurt feelings; rather it means diminishing their power over you.

As you make decisions regarding interactions with your former flame, ask yourself what would make sense for your future self in this situation. Doing this helps shift from emotional reactivity to deliberate responses; take note of which situations or interactions elicit strong emotional reactions so you can better prepare and develop tailored coping strategies.

Weddings and holidays require extra finesse if you share social circles or children. Planning well in advance, being flexible but firm about boundaries, and creating new traditions without depending on ex-interaction can help smooth these potentially trying times with grace - focus instead on creating positive memories instead of trying to avoid making negative ones!

Today's digital environment requires its own set of strategies for effectively managing an online presence. Think carefully about whether a complete break from social media connections would best serve your needs, or whether mute or restrict features can provide enough distance while maintaining social harmony - remembering that digital distance can promote emotional healing.

Even with your best intentions in place, situations with an ex can sometimes prove challenging. Be wary if interactions that leave you feeling anxious or depressed for days afterwards; your ex consistently violates established boundaries, communication issues between yourself and them cannot be maintained professionally or as necessary, or their presence affects other relationships. Don't hesitate to seek professional guidance, strengthen your support system further, reassess and reinforce boundaries where necessary, or limit contact further if necessary.

Remember, rebuilding relationships with an ex takes time. Your goal shouldn't be to become best friends or pretend the past never happened; rather, the goal should be reaching a place in life where their presence doesn't disturb your peace any longer. Success looks different for everyone:

perhaps being able to attend events without anxiety, maintaining cordial co-parenting relationships without animosity between co-parents, feeling nothing when seeing social media updates from them, or hearing their name without feeling emotionally charged is what defines success for you.

Your definition of a healthy ex-relationship should be unique to you; there's no single solution that works across the board, and what works for one season of life may need to change for another. Most importantly, keep perspective; your ex is just another character in your story, not a protagonist or villain - they were simply part of your journey and should not define who or what your story really is about; your growth, healing, and future are the true protagonists here.

Your journey is underway - one day at a time and interaction by interaction, you are creating a life that serves your highest good, which should be celebrated! Remember: the best revenge isn't living well to prove them wrong - it's living well because it is your right and deserves your appreciation.

The best revenge isn't living well to show them - it's living well because you deserve it. But sometimes, living well gets complicated when your life is still tangled up with theirs in ways that go far beyond emotions. Let's talk about how to handle that.

When It's Not Just You: Breaking Up With Added Complications

Have you made it past the initial shock and tear-filled stage, and begun thinking about dating again? But hold up; there's that small matter of an apartment lease you both signed, the dog you share custody for, and Netflix account using their cousin's password - welcome to modern breakups where heartache doesn't simply end when two hearts go separate ways.

Let's be real - breaking up would be so much simpler if it involved simply blocking numbers and burning photos, but in today's complex relationships, relationships create webs of connections that are far harder to untangle than last year's Christmas lights. You aren't just grieving the loss of a partner; you also must navigate an intricate system of shared subscriptions, determine who keeps whom in their friend group, and decide whether it's acceptable to still wish your ex mother happy birthday on Facebook!

At first, sharing living space can be daunting: there's nothing quite as disorienting as having to divide possessions with someone who was once your partner in every way, such as negotiating who gets which item - coffee maker for instance - like it's some high-stakes diplomatic summit! Not to mention your name still remaining on the lease for at least six more months or the security deposit return being as likely as your ex recanting their previous accusations about you!

Financial entanglements? Uh oh. The bank accounts that were opened with great optimism now feel like an elaborate joke from the universe; trying to disentangle your subscriptions from theirs and untangle phone plans while trying to figure out who actually bought that fancy blender you got for Christmas is like operating blindfolded; any mistake could cause havoc and derail the relationship altogether.

No one ever warned us that sharing pets would be such an emotionally-charged topic! Deciding who gets custody of Mr. Whiskers could become far more contentious than any argument over who should do the dishes! Your furry companion doesn't understand why their humans don't live together anymore, and trying to explain concepts such as custody arrangements to an inebriated golden retriever would only increase confusion further.

Extended family situations add an additional layer of complexity. Your ex's mother still likes all your Instagram posts and their little sister sends memes; and it is unclear whether to pretend these relationships never existed or somehow maintain them without making things awkward - it feels like being stuck in relationship limbo where all rules and points don't matter anymore.

Talking of family, there's that small detail of an upcoming family wedding where you were supposed to be a bridesmaid or holiday traditions you have been participating in for years that you no longer are part of - no longer just losing a partner but an entire secondary family with inside jokes, secret recipes, and that eccentric uncle who always liked you more than your ex partner anyway.

So much for shared friend groups: it can be like walking on eggshells trying to figure out who gets custody of which friends, who is invited to what events, and how best to maintain relationships without appearing as though one side is taking sides. Group chat has become a diplomatic minefield; planning even something as basic as birthday dinner requires more planning than military operations!

Assure yourself: Deep breath. Yes, this may seem complicated and overwhelming at times; but know this: step by step you will navigate this challenge with grace (or at least without major public meltdowns) and emerge stronger and wiser on the other side.

Let's begin with the practical aspects, since having a plan can often make emotional hurdles easier to surmount. Living arrangements: whether it's sharing an apartment, co-owning a house together or simply trying to decide who gets to keep that special coffee table you both covet, the key is treating each relationship like a business transaction - keeping an inventory of everything shared, including furniture and kitchen gadgets; be fair but firm about which items matter to each of you, remembering that material items should never prolong emotional suffering!

Financial entanglements should be addressed as soon as possible, which begins by creating an inventory of all shared accounts, subscriptions, and financial commitments (even ones you forgot about like gym memberships!). Draw up a timeline for untangling these accounts; and don't hesitate to seek professional assistance as a financial advisor or mediator can often prove invaluable in doing this without creating unnecessary friction between partners.

Remember when dealing with shared pets that your fur babies need stability just as much as you. Instead of treating pet custody as a contest between two people, approach it from their wellbeing's standpoint instead. Consider factors like work schedules and living situations along with who can provide proper financial means. It is acceptable to create a "pet custody schedule", just make sure that it is done more maturely than your ex partner would prefer.

Family ties can be particularly complex. Relationships you have forged with an ex's family don't need to end just because your romantic relationship did; instead they should evolve. Give yourself permission to maintain meaningful connections that feel authentic but be wary of overstepping boundaries; an occasional text or social media exchange is fine - just maybe for now skip weekly family dinners altogether.

Friendship groups require an artful balance between openness and grace. Be clear with your closest friends about your needs and boundaries without forcing them into choosing sides; rather, focus on nurturing relationships that make you feel supported and understood, being accepting when friends need to maintain connections with both of you simultaneously.

Technology and social media require special care, so take an inventory of all your digital connections - shared cloud storage, streaming services, family phone plans and any other tech connections you share - before devising a plan to separate these services without harming your credit score or losing all your carefully curated playlists. Remember: just because they can still see your Instagram stories doesn't mean you should!

Allow yourself the freedom to be selective when it comes to social obligations and future events, including wedding parties and holiday traditions. A destination wedding where both of you were supposed to be part of the bridal party? Have an honest discussion with the couple to see whether your presence would create unnecessary tension. And this may even be an ideal opportunity to start new traditions that better reflect who you are moving forward.

One essential thing to keep in mind when making decisions involving separation and divorce: reaching out for help isn't just okay - it's essential. From hiring a mediator to help divide assets to consulting with a therapist for emotional processing or simply leaning on friends who've experienced similar scenarios, support is crucial - don't try and tackle all this alone!

Document everything. Keep records of agreements made, expenses shared, and arrangements made - not because things will inevitably go wrong, but so that clarity helps prevent future complications. Use co-parenting apps to schedule pet custody schedules, get agreements written down and save important communications; future you will thank past you for being so organized!

Be mindful that unravelling your life from someone else's is a gradual process, not an event. Some days will pass without incident while on other days you might find yourself crying your eyes out in the pet food aisle as you purchase your ex's favorite treats for their dog - both reactions are perfectly acceptable and completely normal.

Step by step is key to making changes happen - today could be when you cancel that shared Netflix account; tomorrow could bring division of kitchen appliances; next week could see you searching for your own apartment - small steps forward are still steps forward and all add up!

Remember this: any difficult situation you're navigating teaches you something useful about yourself. Perhaps you are learning how to advocate for your needs, set healthy boundaries or navigate complex emotional terrain with grace - skills which will serve you well in all future relationships.

Your task of ending a relationship and disentangling every aspect of it from each other requires work, so if it feels daunting at times or you don't have all of the answers immediately it's okay; some days all you can manage may be choosing who gets to keep throw pillows.

Trust that in time, all these complications will be ironed out. Your lease agreement or issue will come to an end or resolution; pets will adjust to their new schedule; friend groups will find new normals; and most importantly - YOU! - will emerge stronger, wiser and more capable than ever before.

Truth be told: you aren't simply surviving a breakup - rather, you are learning how to navigate complex adult situations with grace and dignity (most of the time), which should make you proud even on those difficult days when patience seems like its waneing.

Keep going, brave soul. Take each challenge as it comes, knowing that you're not alone in finding solutions. In fact, let me share some stories of those who've travelled this path before you; people who've not just endured difficult breakups but used them to forge extraordinary transformations in themselves and in others.

Stories of Resilience: When Heartbreak Becomes a Superpower

Ready? We are in for an emotional ride! These tales won't give you platitudes such as "everything happens for a reason", rather they tell stories from real people who faced their pain head on and decided to turn it into their personal superpower.

Breakups don't just tell sad tales: they tell epic ones in which our hero (that would be you, by the way) emerges victorious from their failed relationship like a Phoenix with stunning hair and an awesome playlist.

Healing can be an uphill struggle. Like riding a rollercoaster through a haunted house, its journey is marked with unexpected twists, jump scares, and moments when it feels as if your lunch might fly right out the window - yet at its heart lies self-discovery, transformation and becoming your greatest self.

Grab some tissues, some ice cream and wine (we don't judge), and let's hear some stories that demonstrate resilience is not about being perfect; rather it is about celebrating each messy and beautiful step along your journey as being part of what makes life meaningful and beautiful.

Meet Kate: Her five-year relationship didn't simply end - it collapsed with the dramatic flair of a Michael Bay film. It turned out her long term partner had been leading an unexpected double life that even the seasoned soap opera writer would find hard to stomach.

Kate discovered the truth like something out of a spy thriller - with hidden phones, credit cards and lies so intricate it was like macrame gone wrong. Most would have crumbled under such betrayal but not Kate; she had resilience that set her apart.

Kate had always been there when needed - with wine in hand, shoulder to cry on, and an abundance of dark humor when things got tough. She was known as the queen of care packages and master at turning tears into laughter; little did she realize these abilities would become her greatest advantage in life.

Kate had an epiphany while struggling through heartbreak: why couldn't she turn her skill for emotional support into a business and develop products to help others navigate heartbreak with more grace (and humor) than herself?

Enter: Resilience Box. Part care package and part survival kit, Kate's boxes provided much-needed comfort during tough times. She included options for the "I can't get out of bed" stage of grieving - including cozy socks, tea, a journal for recording 3am feelings; boxes to help those ready to burn my ex's stuff such as matches, miniature Zen gardens, stress balls for squeezing instead of screaming; as well as boxes with cute undies, confidence-boosting affirmation cards, and gift certificates towards new haircuts (because nothing says "I'm over it!" quite so effectively).

Kate was thrilled by the response she received - it turns out there are lots of people out there in need of extra TLC (and laughter) while getting over their breakups. Kate's business took off faster than her ex's new relationship did! In fact, she started hosting "Resilience Retreats", weekend getaways designed specifically to assist brokenhearted individuals - complete with yoga, wine tasting and bonfire rituals where people could safely burn letters written to former flames (using proper fire safety precautions of course!).

Kate found comfort in helping others heal as she helped herself. Every grateful customer email, hug at retreats or "you got this, girl" message sent over Instagram served as reminders that she could overcome any setback or breakdown.

Dane seemed to have it all in life: great job, friends, and relationship - so when his wife of ten years decided to leave him for her yoga instructor (cliche!) it felt as if someone had pulled the rug out from underneath him completely.

At first, Dane did what many do in response to such heartache: he fell apart. He spent weeks lying on his couch eating delivery pizza and whiskey while sporting an eye-rolling beard worthy of Tom Hanks from Cast Away; playing sad songs over and over until even his dog noticed something amiss.

Dane eventually noticed something was amiss - perhaps it was hearing "All By Myself" for the hundredth time on his breakup playlist, or realizing his beard was becoming its own ecosystem - something was changing and decided it was time for change. He decided it was time to move forward with something different.

He started small. He took a shower, shaved his beard (RIP old friend), went for a stroll around his neighborhood, and even surprised himself by signing up for yoga class!

Dane wasn't exactly known for being the type of man to take risks and dive headlong into something unfamiliar, yet something about the act of confronting his fears, doing the very thing which had driven his wife away, felt like an act of resilience.

But that was true - Dane struggled through his first class, falling out of tree pose more often than desired, and thinking his instructor may have been laughing at his attempts at warrior pose. Yet, class after class he continued coming back until gradually he began to feel himself again.

But Dane didn't stop there; he quickly began exploring other new hobbies - rock climbing, salsa dancing and even improv comedy (talk about confronting fears!). Each new activity felt like a reminder that he could do much more than expected.

One day it dawned on him: What if he could help other people rediscover themselves as well? Could his pain turn into something positive?

Dane began blogging about the journey through heartbreak on his "The Breakup Diaries," his blog-turned-book-turned-community. He shared his own journey in all its stark reality; from good times and bad. Dane interviewed experts from healing to dating to self-care for advice. Additionally, he hosted events - part support group/part dance party - where people could come together and celebrate their own resilience.

Dane soon realized the lesson it could teach him: healing doesn't involve returning to who you were prior to the breakup; rather, it involves becoming someone new - stronger, wiser and more authentically yourself.

Jenna's breakup story is something out of a rom-com nightmare. Imagine: it's her birthday and she expects that her three-year boyfriend to propose; instead, all she gets in response is an awkward text message saying they couldn't make it tonight but decided we should break up instead."

Boom. Mic drop.

Jenna was left reeling. She spent the entire evening of her birthday alone, alternately between crying and scrolling through his Instagram feed (which already featured pictures of his new girlfriend - ouch!).

But then something incredible happened: Jenna woke up the following morning feeling empowered and determined not to allow this situation define her anymore. Looking into her mirror she told herself "The hell with this; this won't define me any longer!"

She started by creating a list of things she had always wanted to try, but had been too afraid (or too busy being in relationships) to take action on them. Skydiving? Done; backpacking through Europe solo? Check; taking pole dancing classes? All set.

Jenna became a woman on a mission. She saved up money from her job as a graphic designer, sold any belongings that wouldn't fit in a backpack and purchased one-way tickets to Barcelona. Over the next year she travelled around crossing items off of her bucket list like never before: danced until dawn in Berlin nightclubs; learned surfing in Bali; volunteered at an elephant sanctuary in Thailand - documenting all this on Instagram which quickly garnered a following inspired by her fearless spirit.

But Jenna's journey was more than simply about fleeing her heartbreak; it was also about rediscovering herself. Between adventures, she engaged in some serious soul searching - journaling, meditation and having long discussions with fellow travellers about life, love and the pursuit of happiness were among many strategies she utilized in an attempt to rediscover herself. Slowly but surely she began healing - not by forgetting her ex but rather by falling back in love with herself again.

Jenna returned home a changed woman. She was confident, self-assured, and radiating with inner peace that only comes from facing your fears and living your truth. She launched a life coaching business helping other women discover resilience and adventure for themselves; plus she felt ready to date again on her terms.

Resilience means different things for every individual; some find purpose in turning pain into purpose, like Dane with his Breakup Diaries; for others it means facing fears and pursuing their dreams like Jenna in her solo travel adventures; for yet others still, resilience means finding humor and heart even after experiencing heartbreak, like Kate with her Resilience Boxes.

Resilience can manifest itself in different forms; no matter the shape it takes. Resilience always boils down to making one choice: choosing yourself. Rising back up when life knocks you down; loving yourself even when no one else seems to; believing your story won't end just because one chapter closed.

Here's the secret: you are the author of your own life story. You get to choose how you show up in the world, love others and live.

No doubt some chapters may bring pain and heartache, leading to ugly crying in the bathroom floor. Yet others will bring joy, laughter, and love - the kind that allows you to conquer the world, starting by loving yourself first.

Attitude is everything; here's to those with strong resolve, to hearts that keep beating even after they've been broken, to spirits that keep shining even during dark times and, most of all, to YOU - who write the narrative for your own epic tales.

Keep writing those chapters, keep turning those pages. Your story has only just begun; and soon enough it'll become a bestseller!

Now let's talk about emotional intelligence (EQ). While it might sound like something from a self-help book from the 90s, trust me - this stuff is legit and it could become your secret weapon in love (and life!).

First things first: emotional intelligence doesn't involve becoming some unfeeling zen master who never feels any negative emotions - that would simply not be possible or healthy! Instead, emotional intelligence means learning the language of both your own heart as well as that of other's hearts.

Imagine learning a foreign language - initially all sounds are gibberish, yet with practice comes understanding its subtle nuances and meanings behind each word. With each passing week and practice comes understanding these nuanced messages from your body and how best to react in each situation.

Emotional intelligence (EQ) is like this for feelings. It involves learning to recognize and name your emotions in order to comprehend where they come from and understand why they surfaced in the first place. Furthermore, developing empathy and intuition so you can read between the lines when someone else speaks is key as well.

At its heart lies emotional intelligence - an acquired skill like any language. All it requires to develop it further is self-awareness, curiosity, and an acceptance that growth rarely comes easily.

So where should you begin? With yourself. Before beginning to read other people's emotional cues, it is crucial that you become adept in reading your own emotions first.

That means being honest with yourself daily, checking in with both your heart and head - asking the tough questions: "What am I feeling right now, why am I feeling it, and what lies beneath this emotion?

Journaling can be an invaluable asset when it comes to emotional well being, but you don't want Instagram-worthy bullet journals - what you need are words from your subconscious mind, unfiltered and stream-of-consciousness writing that may cause some cringe when read back; yet also feels cleansing when read back out loud.

Put pen (or fingers to keyboard) to paper (or fingers to keyboard), and simply let the words come pouring out of you. Don't worry about spelling or grammar or making sense - just get everything out. You might be amazed by what comes pouring out - old wounds, hidden fears and long buried desires could emerge - this is exactly the type of subconscious material we want to uncover; those thoughts driving your actions and reactions all this time!

Once you are comfortable in your own emotional landscape, it's time to explore those of others by setting some limits and boundaries.

Boundaries may sound restrictive at first, but trust me - they're actually essential for healthy relationships. Boundaries act like walls to your emotional home - keeping the good stuff inside while keeping out any unwanted elements that might otherwise invade.

So what do healthy boundaries look like? They mean being aware of your own needs and desires, communicating them clearly (and politely) to others, saying no when necessary and yes when appropriate and honoring your feelings even when they make others uncomfortable.

Establishing boundaries may take practice (and some awkward conversations). But it's well worth your while; by setting clear boundaries, you create space for genuine and authentic connections - the kind that feels safe, supportive, and real.

Emotional intelligence is all about building deeper, more meaningful connections - with yourself and with others.

At its heart, it means learning to articulate your truth without wavering, even when speaking through tears or discomfort. It means cultivating the courage to have tough conversations about issues that matter to you; own up to your mistakes when necessary and apologize when someone's been injured unintentionally.

Empathy and compassion are essential in becoming an excellent listener, friend, and partner. By tuning into another person's world with empathy and compassion you will experience their pain as if it were your own.

Yes, emotional intelligence can be difficult. There may be days where it all seems easy and effortless; other days might leave you questioning how best to "regulate your emotions" when things feel too much for you.

Healing isn't a linear process; rather, it's an ongoing journey filled with twists and turns and unexpected detours and pit stops. To stay on the journey successfully and show up for yourself at all times (especially during challenging moments). The key is not giving up when things get tough - keeping going, even on difficult days (and especially then).

Attracting healthier relationships becomes much simpler as you develop emotional intelligence and learn to love and accept yourself more fully.

Because this is how it works: what we attract is who we are. When we act with emotional intelligence and tap into both our own hearts and those of others, we start attracting individuals who share similar views; people who respect our boundaries, acknowledge our feelings, and appreciate us for who we truly are.

That, my friend, is the ultimate goal: not simply healing from heartbreak (though that's important too), but becoming someone who attracts love, joy and abundance into their life - someone with strong emotional intelligence who radiates positive vibes like a meteor shower.

Continue doing the work; remain curious about yourself; set boundaries and have difficult discussions; practice empathy and kindness even when it's hard; don't stop now!

As is often the case, learning to love yourself will lead to loving others more fully. Acceptance of oneself leads to acceptance of all. And showing up for yourself allows others to do the same.

Life is about showing up, being present, loving hard and living fully - that is its meaning! Here's to you and your emotional intelligence journey; may the lessons be with you and may love flourish.

Continue to illuminate the world. Now more than ever it needs a beacon like you.

Plot Twist- You're the Main Character

Welcome to the end of our journey, when we can take a step back and consider the big picture. If this book were a movie, this would be where the music builds as the camera pans over the horizon, showing how far we have travelled together.

Here's the surprising twist: this story wasn't ever about your ex, it was always about you - even when it felt like your role had been reduced to "sad ex #2."

Breakups often leave us feeling powerless, as though our roles were secondary in someone else's drama. Yet, remember this experience has given you an opportunity to step into the spotlight and rewrite your narrative.

Think back: when was the last time you truly were the star of your own life? When was the last time that decisions were based solely on what YOU wanted without considering anyone else's needs and opinions? When was the last time that selfishness meant prioritizing YOUR happiness and growth first?

Like me, relationships often force us to compromise and consider someone else's wants and dreams alongside our own. That doesn't have to be seen as bad - in fact it can help create strong partnerships - but in doing so we may lose sight of our individual paths altogether.

That is where singlehood comes into its own: as an opportunity to rediscover who you are when not part of a couple, and to fall in love with yourself all over again without apology or regrets.

As much as it may feel like punishment right now, starting over could actually be the greatest blessing in disguise! Give it time - maybe something better comes along?

What if this breakup was the catalyst you needed to finally pursue that dream you have been postponing, or take that solo trip you've always talked about, or sign up for that class that intimidated you? Maybe this is your opportunity to step outside your comfort zone and experience new ways of being courageous while discovering who and what lies within you?

Growth is never an easy journey, and I know you may feel uncomfortable as your world changes around you. On some days you may wish for things to return back the way they were; having that familiar and comforting sense that comes from being part of a couple. Other nights might feel lonely or scary; when it seems as if no one will hold you and tell you it will all work out okay.

But here's the thing - no one needs to tell you this; you can be your own source of comfort and reassurance, holding your own hand when things become challenging, offering words of support when things look grim, becoming the hero in your own story and saving yourself again and again.

Well, who knows? Maybe you'll surprise yourself by discovering just how strong you truly are; by how adaptable and resilient you are when forced to rely on yourself alone for resources; perhaps discovering deeper levels of compassion for both yourself and others who may also be going through struggle; maybe finding that sense of independence and self-sufficiency which you had no idea existed within yourself!

Importantly, though, is the possibility of falling in love with who you become after embarking on this journey - someone who understands their worth, refuses to settle for anything less than they deserve, has courage to pursue their dreams while learning from past errors, and understands heartbreak is simply part of life's story.

Saluting you as the central figure in your own epic tale: to you for being such an unforgettable protagonist; here's to all the unexpected twists, turns and detours that make life rich and unpredictable; here's to heartache that fractures us open, only for healing to restore us all to greater strength than before.

As you step back into the world, I hope that when closing this book and entering its pages for good, a few things remain clear to you: that your worth doesn't depend on whether or not you are currently in a relationship; you are already whole, complete and deserving of love just the way you are; healing isn't linear and that it is okay to experience setbacks, bad days and doubt.

But most importantly, I hope you remember that you are the author of your own story. You get to decide what comes next and design a life you love for yourself - choosing people, experiences and adventures that will shape and challenge you while making you feel alive!

Be brave! Dare to be bold. Embark on adventures without regrets or fear; embrace unexpected turns as stepping stones toward something wonderful you may yet see; know that no matter what occurs, you always had this.

Here lies the final twist of your own story: you are no longer just the main character; instead, you are your own hero: warrior or phoenix rising from ashes - finally coming through and showing yourself as someone worth waiting for all along.

So live your truth, seek joy, spread your wings and fly. And know that wherever your journey leads you are supported by an army of fellow main characters cheering you on all along the way.

Welcome to your new chapter; now let the journey begin!

Thank you for reading "The Break Up - Your Lifeline Through the Absolute Dumpster Fire of Heartbreak!" If this book helped you navigate the tough waters of heartbreak, made you laugh when you thought you couldn't, or simply reminds you that you're not alone, I'd be grateful if you'd share your experience with others. Your **Amazon review** could help someone else find the support they need during their own breakup journey. A few words about what resonated with you or how the book supported your healing would mean the world. Thank you for letting me be part of your story!

Printed in Dunstable, United Kingdom

65501811R00087